PEGAN DIET FACTS A

Find out All You Need to Know about the Pegan Diet

Plus 30 Healthy & Most Delicious Recipes for Weight Loss,

Blood Sugar Control and Diabetes

Shelly Herkel

Disclaimer and Terms of Use

Effort has been made to ensure that the information in this book is accurate and complete, however, the author and the publisher do not warrant the accuracy of the information, text and graphics contained within the book due to the rapidly changing nature of science, research, known and unknown facts and internet. The Author and the publisher do not hold any responsibility for errors, omissions or contrary interpretation of the subject matter herein. This book is presented solely for motivational and informational purposes only.

Table of Contents

INTRODUCTION

The Pegan Diet is a new diet that combines Vegan and Paleo Diets. Mark Hyman, a nutritionist and doctor, discovered this diet last year which has proved so far that is very helpful indeed; not to mention that it is becoming popular day after day. Many thanks to its varied benefits that help you in more than one way.

The best thing about this diet is that is combines and balances the best of the 2 famous diets Paleo and Vegan; which means that it provides you with double benefits that no other diet can give you.

This diet is one of a kind because it is so cheap and easy to follow, as it also does not make you follow so many complicated rules like other diets. Everything about it is clear and easy to do, not to mention that the benefits that this diet provides your body with are countless and very important.

The Pegan Diet is not focused only on losing weight as some of you might think, as it actually about improving your body and making it healthy from the inside and outside at the same time.

The Pegan Diet so far is the best diet in the world, as it makes you achieve a healthy body and brain faster, without wasting any more time or money. Grownups or youngsters, everybody can follow this diet without an exception.

To make your journey easier, we offer you in this book all the information as well as answers to almost all the questions that you might ask about this diet as well as the most mouth-watering recipes that you can start your journey towards the Pegan Diet with.

Tighten your seat belts and get ready to dive in the depths of the Pegan Diet and see for yourself how it can make your life much more wonderful.

Enjoy the ride.

WHAT IS THE PEGAN DIET?

Throughout the years and especially in the 21 century, our world has known so many changes and developments in all domains including food and diets.

After noticing the struggle that so many people have because of their weight and how much it impacts their lives, especially knowing that losing weight has been a very difficult task; the nutrition experts have discovered throughout the years many healthy and different diets to lose weight and maintain a healthy body, on top of their list there is the Paleo and the Vegan diets that a large percentage of people have found to be very helpful.

After so many tests and researches, experts have discovered a perfect equation that helps to get rid of excess weight faster and keeps your body healthy and perfect. Not to mention that it is not only for losing weight but overall for maintaining a healthy lifestyle and body at the same time.

This equation surprisingly integrates and balances completely two different diets into one; which are the Vegan diet and Paleo diet.

Doctor Mark Hayman, the public health expert and New York Times bestselling author has managed to bring to the light this new diet called « **Pegan** » that have managed so far to give amazing results.

This Diet is mainly about 75 % of plants and 25 % of meat and vegetarian protein, but it does not include dairy products.

Overall, Pegan Diet combines all kinds of foods that your body is in need of such as good cholesterol, grains, and proteins but at the same time avoids all the bad and unhealthy foods.

WHAT THE EXPERTS ARE SAYING ABOUT THE PEGAN DIET AND ITS BENEFITS?

Many international nutrition experts around the world have recommended the Pegan Diet. One of them is Susie Burrell, one of Australia's leading dieticians, a resident dietician on a weekly radio segment with, Consultant Dietician at Sydney University Sport, Body Science International, Go Natural Foods, Peppercorn Food Company and SIMPLE skincare.

Susie Burrell said to the Daily Mail Australia "A Pegan Diet mixes the principles of Paleo while incorporating more fibre and grains, adding to a more fibre-rich diet overall,"

Since the Pegan Diet is originally a combination of 2 diets, you can automatically know that its benefits are doubled and effective. To state the benefits of this diet, will need a whole new book but here are some few benefits that you should know of:

- **Weight Loss:**
  The majority of people choose to go on a diet that helps them lose weight and what is better than the Pegan Diet.
  This diet encourages you to eat lot of plant, which makes you lose weight fast and easily as it also gives your body more fibers, antioxidants and many other vitamins that sustains and offer your body the energy that it needs.

- **Healthier Skin:**
  Pegan Diet is rich in fibers and fats that keep your skin healthy and perfect; which reflects on your whole appearance and gives you a 100 % natural glow without having to use any products.

- **Cleanse Body Organs:**
  Throughout our everyday life and routine, our bodies do not only consume what we eat or drink only but what we smell and touch as well. We might not pay attention to it, but the toxics in the air that we breathe are more than enough to cause us so many chronic and dangerous diseases. The Pegan Diet equips our bodies with enough antidotes and different vitamins to stand against these toxics and clean our body organs as well from the inside.

- **Cheap:**
  Thanks to the Pegan Diet, you will save a lot of money without even realizing it. This diet is about eating lots of veggies and fruits, so whenever there is a sale on a specific ingredient buy this in bulk and freeze.

  In no time, you will find yourself with enough supplements for a year or more, which will cover your needs and save you a huge amount of money.

- **Stand Against Chronic Diseases:**
  Most of the chronic diseases are triggered by the high stress and our poor if not choices dietaries and lifestyles; which lead to chronic inflammation that lead as well to chronic diseases.
  The Pegan Diet and lifestyle shield your body with antioxidants, vitamins and minerals that fight and protect your body from these inflammations.

- **Double Benefits:**
  As you already know, the Pegan Diet is result of combining Vegan and Paleo diets; which means that you will get the benefits of both diets by following one.

WHAT TO EAT ON THE PEGAN DIET

The foods that you can eat for Pegan Diet are similar to an extent to what you eat on Vegan or Paleo diets, but it is more focused on the Vegan diet.

- Eat foods that are full of proteins and the good fats such as:
    1. Avocado
    2. Coconut
    3. Nuts
    4. Seeds
    5. Sardines
    6. Olive oil
    7. Lentils
    8. Animal meats
    9. Gluten-free whole grains
    10. Veggies
    11. Fruits
- Stay away from soybeans oil, canola, corn and sunflower oil because they contain lot of calories; you can use instead omega 3 fats.

- Avoid all dairy products, gluten, starchy beans and sugar.

In this diet, you have to focus mainly on veggies and fruits; 75 % of your meals must consist of veggies and fruits whereas you can eat meat only as a condiment not as a main course.

IS THE PEGAN DIET BETTER THAN THE PALEO OR VEGAN DIETS?

Many of you wonder why Pegan Diet is better than Paleo and Vegan diet. Here is a list of the negative and positive elements in each diet, so that you can see for yourself why Pegan Diet is the best.

Paleo Diet:
Paleo diet or in other words the caveman life style focuses on making you eat like our ancestors used to. It is based on consuming lots of meat, veggies, fruits, healthy oils and some limited types of seeds.

Pros: Just like Vegan and Pegan Diets, this diet helps you lose weight, lower diseases and allergies as well; makes your muscles and brain healthier as it also helps maintain a healthy body.

Cons: The worst thing about this diet is that it makes you eat huge amounts of meat, which might not be so healthy after all. Not to mention that it is expensive, you have to spend a lot of money on meat.

Vegan Diet:
In Vegan diet, you can eat only organic products and foods; you have to stay away from dairy products, honey, and any kind of meat, eggs and anything that uses some of these products such as cosmetics etc.

Pros: This diet is absolutely healthy as it lowers the risk of heart diseases and the most of all helps you to lose weight as it also improves longevity. The best thing about this diet is that it is cheap and will not only help you maintain a healthy body but save a lot of money.

Cons: This diet is completely free from any kind of meat, although it is very healthy but this diet makes you to miss many vitamins that meat gives you such as vitamins B12, B3, B6, Iron, Zinc, Selenium and so many other different minerals and vitamins.

Pegan Diet:
This diet combines the best of the Vegan and Paleo Diets, as it focuses on healthy oils, veggies, fruits, small amount of beans, meat and gluten free grains as well.

Pros: This diet offers you exactly the pros of Vegan and Paleo Diets at the same time.

Cons: Since the Pegan Diet has combined only the best of the Paleo and Vegan diet, they are no cons to mention right now.

TIPS FOR A PEGAN LIFESTYLE

Pegan Diet is super easy, so it does not require a lot of tips or instructions. The only 5 tips that you will need are:

- **Stay away from sugar:**
  Once you decide to go on the Pegan Diet, you have to keep in your mind that you will not be able to eat sugar. You can just eat it as a treat from time to time with a small amount.

- **Vary your meat recourse:**
  Do not concentrate on a specific type of meat, try to vary it from time to time and use it only as a side dish.

- **Consume lots of veggies and fruits:**
  Fill your everyday meals and main courses with different and lots of veggies and fruits. Use colorful veggies and fruits to encourage yourself.

- **Look for good fats:**
  Consume healthy oils, avocado, nuts and seeds to fulfill your body with the good fats that it needs.

- **Stay away from dairy products:**
  Stay away from any dairy products; otherwise you will ruin your diet completely.

THE PEGAN DIET RULES

The pegan does not actually require a lot of rules, there are overall 5 simple rules that you can consider. To make your diet more efficient and lucrative, you can simply follow those easy and helpful 5 rules.

1. Use Meat as a condiment:

Try to vary your meat sources and use them with small amounts in your side dishes only. This method helps you benefit from the vitamins that meat has to offer, and at the same time prevent you from its disadvantages.

2. Eat small amount of beans:

As much as beans are full of vitamins and many other benefits, a lot of people complain of bloating and digestives problems. To prevent this, avoid starchy beans and try to not exceed half cup of beans a day, if you want to use it.

3. Gluten free grains are the best:

Quinoa, rice and oats are one of the best sources of fibers, so make sure to include half cup of gluten free grains in your everyday meals.

4. Eat 2 eggs a day:

Eggs play an important role in the Pegan Diet. You need to eat 2 eggs for breakfast or sometime in the day, because they provide you with many minerals, vitamins as well as healthy and good fats.

5. Dairy products:

Avoid and do not go near dairy products at all, because they have proven that they damage our bodies more then they help it.

QUICK AND EASY PEGAN DIET RECIPES

BREAKFAST RECIPES

Baked Eggs with Avocado

Serves: 4

Ingredients:

- 2 avocados cut into half lengthwise
- 4 eggs
- 1 tablespoon of chopped chives
- Black pepper
- Salt

Directions:

1. Scoop out 2 tablespoons from the avocado to make more space then place them on a baking sheet.

2. Crack each egg and put each in half avocado and season them with some salt and pepper.

3. Preheat the oven on 425 F and bake them for 15 to 20 minutes.

4. Serve warm and enjoy.

Calories: 449

Mini Eggs Muffins

Serves: 4

Ingredients:

- 4 eggs
- Half cup of chopped zucchinis
- 1/3 cup of milk
- 1/6 cup of chopped red bell pepper
- 1 tablespoon and half of chopped onion
- 4 ounces of shredded goat cheese
- Salt
- Pepper

Directions:

1. In a bowl, mix the eggs with milk and season with some salt and pepper then add the rest of the ingredients and mix them well.

2. Preheat the oven on 350 f and bake them for 15 to 20 minutes.

3. Once the time is up, serve and enjoy.

Calories: 206

Veggies and Eggs Casserole

Serves: 5

Ingredients:

- 5 ounces of hash browns
- 1/2 cup of cooked and diced ham
- 1 /2cup and half of shredded goat cheese
  1/4 cup of sliced mushrooms
- 1/4 cup of skim water
- 4 eggs
- 1/8 cup of chopped green pepper
- 1/8 of chopped onion
- Salt
- Pepper

Directions:

1. In a greased baking dish, layer the hash browns then layer half of the cheese on top of it followed by ham, mushroom, onion and pepper.

2. In a bowl, whisk the eggs with water and season with some salt and pepper as well as the rest of the cheese.

3. Poor the egg mix on top of the veggies then bake it for 20 to 30 minutes on 350 F.

4. Serve it warm and enjoy.

Calories: 88

Avocado Tacos

Serves: 4

Ingredients:

- 2 eggs
- 1 small handful of torn cilantro
- 1 chopped potato
- 4 corn tortillas
- 1 sliced avocado
- 1/2 teaspoon of garlic powder
- 1/2 teaspoon of onion powder
- 1 tablespoon of olive oil
- Salt
- Pepper

Directions:

1. In a large bowl, mix the eggs with garlic powder, a pinch of salt and pepper then cook it in a skillet with olive oil.

2. In a baking dish, mix onion powder with the chopped potato and season it with a pinch of salt and pepper.

3. Preheat the oven on 400 F and bake it for 15 minutes.

4. Place the cooked eggs on the tortillas followed by the potatoes, avocado and cilantro then wrap them.

5. Serve it and enjoy.

Calories: 221

Oat Bowl and Vanilla

Serves: 2

Ingredients:

- ¾ cup of rolled oats
- 2 cups of unsweetened coconut water
- ½ cup of dry fruits
- 2 tablespoons of nuts
- 1 teaspoon of vanilla extract
- 1 teaspoon of honey
- ½ teaspoon of cinnamon

Directions:

1. Bring the coconut water to a boil then add to it the rolled oats and cinnamon with vanilla and allow to cook from 15 to 20 minutes on low heat.

2. Once the time is up, allow it to rest with the cover on for 5 minutes then pour it in the serving bowls and top it with the rest of the ingredients.

3. Enjoy.

Calories: 721

LUNCH RECIPES

Swiss Chard and Chick Peas Patties

Serves: 2 to 3

Ingredients:

- 4 cups of chopped Swiss chard
- 15 ½ ounces of chick peas
- 3 tablespoons of oat flour
- 4 tablespoons of olive oil
- 3 chopped cloves of garlic
- 1 tablespoon and half of lemon juice
- 1 tablespoon and half of tahini
- Salt
- Black pepper
- ¼ teaspoon of cumin

Directions:

1. In a food processor, blend the Swiss chard with lemon juice, garlic, cumin, chick peas, tahini, a pinch of salt and pepper until they become smooth.

2. Pour the mix into a large bowl then add to it the flour gradually and mix it well.

3. Shape the mix into medium patties then cook it in a heated skillet with olive oil for 1 to 2 minutes on each side.

4. Serve them right away with some garlic sauce and enjoy.

Calories: 154

Sweet Potato Wraps

Serves: 6

Ingredients:

- 2 cups of chopped sweet potatoes
- 1 chopped onion
- 1 chopped red bell pepper
- 12 corn tortillas
- 3 cups of enchilada sauce
- 15 ounces of black beans
- 1 cup of cooked and shredded turkey
- 2 minced cloves of garlic
- 1 tablespoon of lime juice
- 1 tablespoon of olive oil
- 1 teaspoon of chilli powder
- 1/2 teaspoon of cumin
- Salt

Directions:

1. Bring the potatoes with some water to a boil in a saucepan then reduce the heat and allow it to simmer for 5 minutes.

2. Once the time is up, drain it and set it aside.

3. Sauté the garlic with onion and olive oil in a large skillet for 5 minutes then add to them the shredded turkey and season with salt and pepper.

4. Allow to cook for another 5 minutes then add the beans with pepper and potatoes then cook for another 8 minutes.

5. Once the time is up, turn off the heat and add the lime juice with cumin, chilli powder and half cup of the enchilada sauce as well.

6. In a greased baking dish, spread the rest of the enchilada sauce.

7. Divide the potato sauce on the corn tortillas and wrap them then place them in the baking dish on top of the sauce.

8. Preheat the oven on 350 F and bake them for 20 minutes.

7. Serve it hot and enjoy.

Calories: 549

Stuffed Sweet Potatoes

Serves: 2

Ingredients:

- 1 bunch of kale
- 1 can of black beans
- 2 sweet potatoes
- 1 tablespoon of olive oil
- 1 minced clove of garlic
- Salt

Directions:

1. Poke the sweet potatoes well with a fork then place them on a baking sheet and bake them for 45 to 50 min on 375 F.

2. In the meantime, heat the olive oil in a skillet and sauté in it the garlic for 1 minute then add it to the kale with 1/3 cup of water.

3. Place the lid on and allow it to cook for 3 minutes, season with some salt and allow to cook for another 15 minutes on low heat.

4. Once the time is up, add the beans and cook them for another 5 minutes and adjust the seasoning.

5. Slice the potato in half lengthwise without cutting completely then fill it with the kale and beans mix and top with your favorite salsa.

6. Serve it warm and enjoy.

Calories: 474

Potato and Lentils Pie

Serves: 6

Ingredients:

- 3 pounds of golden potatoes
- 1 cup and half of uncooked green lentils
- 10 ounces of chopped veggies mix
- 4 cups of veggies broth
- 2 minced cloves of garlic
- 3 tablespoons of Vegan butter
- 2 teaspoons of dry thyme
- Salt
- Pepper

Directions:

1. Slice the potatoes and boil with some water for 20 to 30 minutes.

2. In a large bowl, mash the potato with butter then season it with salt and pepper.

3. In a large sauce pan, sauté the onion with garlic for 5 minutes then add to it the lentils, veggies broth and thyme then bring all to a boil.

4. Adjust the seasoning and lower the heat then allow it to cook until the lentils become tender.

5. Once the lentils become well-cooked add the veggies and allow them to cook for another 10 minutes then add 3 tablespoons of the mashed potato to the mixture.

6. Pour the mixture into a baking dish and top it with a layer of the mashed potato.

7. Preheat the oven on 425 F and bake it for 10 to 15 minutes.

8. Serve it warm and enjoy.

Calories: 396

Veggies Lunch Bowl

Serves: 2

Ingredients:

- 1 julienned zucchini
- 2 julienned carrots
- 1 cup of sliced cabbage
- 3 sliced onions
- 1 sliced red bell pepper
- ¾ cup of frozen edamame
- 1 tablespoon of hemp seeds
- 1 teaspoon of sesame seeds
- 4 tablespoons of pesto sauce

Directions:

1. In a large bowl combine all the ingredients and mix the well.

2. Serve it and enjoy.

Calories: 420

DINNER RECIPES

Chili Lentils Soup

Serves: 6

Ingredients:

- 1 cup and half of green lentils
- 4 cups of veggies broth
- 1 diced onion
- 2 minced stalks of lemon grass
- ¼ cup of coconut milk
- 3 tablespoons of lemon juice
- Half teaspoon of turmeric
- 1 tablespoon of grape seeds oil
- Half teaspoon of cinnamon
- Half teaspoon of cardamom
- Salt
- Pepper

Directions:

1. In a large pot, combine the lentils with broth turmeric and thyme, bring them to a boil then lower the heat and allow them to simmer for 20 minutes.

2. In the meantime, sauté the onion with oil for 5 minutes then add to it the rest of the ingredients and cook them for 1 minute.

3. Once the time is up, dump the onion mix into the lentils and adjust the seasoning.

4. Serve it hot and enjoy.

Calories: 420

Zucchini Noodles Soup

Serves: 4

Ingredients:

- 1 cup of baby kale
- 1 cup of coconut milk
- 1 cup of pizza sauce
- 1/2 cup of sliced in half cherry tomatoes
- 2 tablespoons of pine nuts
- 1 tablespoon and half of non-dairy butter
- 5 spiralized yellow squash
- Salt
- Pepper
- 2 teaspoons of chili flakes
- 1 teaspoon of onion powder
- 1 teaspoon of garlic powder

Directions:

1. Combine in large saucepan the milk with oil, garlic, chili, onion, a pinch of salt and pepper then cook and whisk them until they become thick.

2. Add the zucchini noodle and kale into the saucepan and cook them for 3 min.

3. Adjust the seasoning and serve them with pine nuts cherry tomatoes.

4. Enjoy.

Calories: 227

Ratatouille

Serves: 2

Ingredients:

- 1 sliced zucchinis
- 1 sliced squash
- 1 sliced red bell pepper
- 1 sliced eggplant
- ½ cup chopped onion
- 1 cup of tomato purée
- 2 tablespoons of olive oil
- 2 thinly sliced cloves of garlic
- ¼ teaspoon of pepper flakes
- ¼ teaspoon of oregano
- ¼ teaspoon of salt
- Pepper
- 4 chopped sprigs of thyme

Directions:

1. In a baking pan, combine the tomato purée with salt, pepper, onion, 1 tablespoon of olive oil, oregano and pepper flakes, arrange the sliced veggies on top of the sauce.

2. Drizzle the rest of the olive oil on top with the chopped thyme and cover the baking pan with a parchment paper.

3. Preheat the oven on 375 f and bake it for 4 to 55 minutes.

4. Top it with some goat cheese and pepperoni then serve it and enjoy.

Calories: 85

Veggies Pizza

Serves: 2

Ingredients:

- 1 sliced eggplant
- 1 small shredded Italian eggplant
- 2 sliced tomatoes
- 2 sliced yellow zucchinis
- ½ cup of sliced pepperoni
- 1 jumbo egg
- ¼ cup and 2 tablespoons of ground flaxseeds
- 4 tablespoons of almond flour
- 2 tablespoons of olive oil
- Balsamic vinegar
- Pepper
- Salt

Directions:

1. In a large bowl, mix the flaxseeds with almond flour, shredded eggplant, jumbo egg, 1 tablespoon of olive oil, a pinch of salt and pepper until you form a dough.

2. Allow the dough to rest for 5 min then press it into a baking sheet.

3. Preheat the oven on 375 f and bake it for 20 minutes.

4. Once the time is up, arrange the veggies and pepperoni on top of the pizza crust and season them with some salt and pepper.

5. Drizzle some olive oil n top of them then bake them for another 13 minutes.

6. Serve it warm and enjoy.

Calories: 201

Zucchini with Chicken and Arugula

Serves: 4

Ingredients:

- 6 julienned zucchinis
- 3 cups of arugula
- 1 cup of diced chicken
- ¾ cup of water
- ¾ cup of soaked cashews
- 1/3 cup of fresh lemon juice
- 1 tablespoon of Tahiti
- 1 tablespoon of olive oil
- Half teaspoon of grated nutmeg
- 2 cloves of garlic
- Salt
- Pepper

Direction:

1. In a food processor, blend the drained nuts with, tahini, water, garlic, lemon juice and nutmeg until they become smooth.

2. In a skillet cook the chicken with olive oil until it is well done then season it with some salt and pepper and set it aside.

3. In a large bowl, mix all the ingredient together then serve them in enjoy.

Calories: 332

DESSERT RECIPES

Coconut and Cashews Pie Blizzard

Serves: 2 to 3

Ingredients:

- 1 cup of unsweetened coconut milk
- 1 cup of soaked cashews for overnight
- 1 sliced banana
- 5 pitted, soaked in hot water for 10 min drained dates
- 2 tablespoons of ground banana cookies
- 2 tablespoons of melted coconut oil
- 1 teaspoon of vanilla extract

Directions:

1. In a food processor, blend the coconut milk, drained cashews, drained dates, coconut oil and vanilla until they become creamy and smooth.

2. Pour the batter into an ice cube tray then place them in the fridge until it freezes.

3. Divide the ice-cream into 6 portions then fill each serving glass with 1 portion then top it with some slices of banana and ground cookies.

4. Repeat the process to create a second layer.

4. Allow it to chill in the fridge for 1 hour before serving.

Calories: 443

Cacao and Almond Pudding

Serves: 2

Ingredients:

- 1 cup and ¼ of unsweetened almond milk
- ¼ cup of chia seeds
- 3 tablespoons of cacao powder
- 1 tablespoon of raw honey

Directions:

1. In a large jar with a lid, combine all the ingredients and shake them until they are well combined then place it in the fridge for 4 hours or more.

2. Garnish it with some dark chocolate and enjoy.

Calories: 82

Panna cotta Tart

Serves: 4

Ingredients:

- 400 ml of coconut cream
- 100 ml of cream substitute
- 3 tablespoons of ground hazel nuts
- 1 cup and half of ground pecan nuts
- ½ cup of dry and chopped cranberries
- 3 tablespoons of shredded coconut
- 4 tablespoons of coconut oil
- 2 tablespoons of sugar
- 2 tablespoons of cacao powder
- 10 g of gelatin powder
- The zest of 1 lemon

Directions:

1. In a large bowl, combine the pecan nuts with cranberries, shredded coconut, hazelnuts, cacao and coconut oil then press them to the bottom of a greased baking dish and place it in the fridge to chill.

2. In the meantime, heat the coconut cream and substitute in a saucepan then add to it the gelatin and whisk it until it dissolves.

3. Add the lemon zest and sugar then pour it in the mold of the tart and place it in the fridge for 2 hours or more.

4. Garnish it with your favorite toppings and enjoy.

Calories: 619

Vanilla and Chia Seeds Pudding

Serves: 2

Ingredients:

- 1 cup of unsweetened almond milk
- ¼ cup of chia seeds
- 2 tablespoons of maple syrup
- 1 teaspoon of vanilla extract

Directions:

1. In a bowl, combine all the ingredients well and place them in the fridge.

2. Allow them to chill for 4 hours.

3. Once the time is up, garnish it with your favorite toppings and enjoy.

Calories: 48

Cinnamon Rolls with Apple Sauce

Serves: 8 to 10

Ingredients:

- Half cup of coconut flour
- 1/3 cup of apple sauce
- 3 tablespoons of xylitol
- 1 tablespoon of melted non-dairy butter
- 3 packets of stevia
- 2 teaspoons and half of cinnamon
- 2 teaspoons of xantham
- 1 teaspoon of baking powder
- 3 eggs

Directions:

1. In a large bowl, mix the eggs with apple sauce and a pinch of salt then add to them the coconut flour with half teaspoon of cinnamon, xantham and stevia one after another.

2. Knead the dough well for 1 to 2 minutes then roll with roller pin and brush it surface with the melted butter.

3. In a small bowl, combine the rest of the cinnamon and xylitol and sprinkle it on top of the dough.

4. Roll the dough softly and carefully then cut it into 8 to 10 rolls.

5. Preheat the oven on 400 F and bake the rolls for 15 to 20 minutes.

Calories: 238

SNACKS RECIPES

Courgette Sandwiches

Serves: 2

Ingredients:

- 4 zucchinis halved and cut half lengthwise
- 1/2 cup of pizza sauce
- Half cup of sliced cherry tomatoes
- ¼ cup of sliced onion
- ¼ cup of chopped olives
- 2 tablespoons of basil

Directions:

1. Spread 1 tablespoon of pizza sauce on each half of the zucchinis and top it with the sliced onion, olives and cherry tomatoes at last then bake it 20 to 25 minutes on 400 F.

2. Serve them warm and enjoy.

Calories: 131

Eggplants Rolls

Serves: 8 to 12

Ingredients:

- 1 eggplant thinly sliced lengthwise
- 1 zucchini thinly sliced lengthwise
- 8 ounces of cashews soaked and processed with garlic
- 1 teaspoon of coconut oil
- ½ cup of tomato sauce

Directions:

1. Dry the slices of zucchini and eggplant with a paper towel and set them aside.

2. Cook the slices of eggplants and zucchinis with coconut oil in a skillet for 1 to 2 minutes on each side.

3. Place 1 tablespoon of processed cashew in each slice and wrap it then place it on a serving plate.

4. Drizzle tomato sauce on top of them and enjoy.

Calories: 127

Oats and Cereal Bars

Serves: 12

Ingredients:

- ½ cup of organic peanut butter
- ½ cup of maple syrup
- ½ cup of crispy rice cereal
- 1 cup and half of rolled oats
- ½ cup of Vegan unsweetened protein powder
- 3 tablespoons of dark chocolate chips
- 1/2 tablespoon of coconut oil
- 1 teaspoon of vanilla extract

Directions:

1. In a large bowl, mix the dry ingredients and add to them the wet ingredients then roll them, after that cut them into your favorite shapes and place them in a the freezer for 10 to 15 minutes.

2. In the meantime, melt the coconut oil with chocolate until you get a sauce then drizzle it on top of the protein bars.

3. Freeze them for another 15 minutes and enjoy.

Calories: 190

Pumpkin and Almond Squares

Serves: 9

Ingredients:

- 2 cups of gluten free graham crumbs
- ¼ cup of maple syrup
- ¼ cup of coconut milk
- ¼ cup of melted coconut oil
- 2 tablespoons of coconut nectar syrup
- 2 tablespoons of almond milk
- 1 tablespoon and half of arrowroot flour
- 1/2 teaspoon of cinnamon
- 14 ounces of pumpkin purée
- 1/3 cup of natural cane sugar
- ¼ teaspoon of ginger
- ¼ teaspoon of nutmeg

Directions:

1. In a bowl, combine the graham crumbs with melted coconut oil and coconut nectar then press it firmly in the bottom of a greased baking pan to make the crust.

2. Preheat the oven on 350 F and bake it for 10 minutes.

3. In a large bowl, combine the rest of the ingredients and mix them well then place it on top of the crust and bake it for 40 to 43 minutes at 350 F.

4. Once the time is up cut it into squares and place in the fridge to cool down.

5. Garnish it with your favorite toppings and enjoy.

Calories: 344

Pizza Tortillas

Serves: 8

Ingredients:

- 2 tortillas
- 15 ounces of cooked black beans
- ½ cup of chopped onion
- ½ cup of chopped avocado
- 1/2 cup of chopped bell pepper
- 1/3 cup of cheese sauce
- 1/3 cup of pizza sauce
- 3 tablespoons of minced parsley
- Grated non-dairy cheese
- Salt

Directions:

1. In a large bowl, combine the beans with parsley, pepper, onion, cheese sauce and a pinch of salt then mix them well.

2. Place the tortillas on a baking sheet and spread whatever amount of pizza sauce then top it with the beans mix.

3. Sprinkle the grated cheese on top and bake them for 10 minutes on 350 F.

4. Serve them warm and enjoy.

Calories: 254

SMOOTHIES

Green Smoothie

Serves: 3

Ingredients:

- 1 cup of kale leaves
- ½ cup of red grape fruit juice
- 1 chopped sweet apple
- 1 cup of chopped cucumber
- 1/8 cup of mint leaves
- 4 tablespoons of hemp heart
- 4 ice cubes
- ½ cup of chopped celery
- ¼ cup of frozen mango
- ½ tablespoon of coconut oil

Directions:

1. In a food processor, blend all the ingredients then serve your smoothie and enjoy.

Calories: 495

Strawberry and Avocado Smoothie

Serves: 4

Ingredients:

- 1 cup of coconut water
- 4 ice cubes
- ½ avocado
- 1 cup of frozen strawberries
- 1 chopped apple
- 1 chopped beet
- 3 tablespoons of lemon juice

Directions:

1. Put all the ingredients in a blender and blend them well.

2. Serve and enjoy.

Calories: 101

Chia Seeds and Pumpkin Smoothie

Serves: 4

Ingredients:

- 2 cups of almond milk
- 1 frozen banana
- 1 cup of canned pumpkin
- ½ cup of rolled oats
- 2 tablespoons of chia seeds
- 2 tablespoons of maple syrup
- ½ tablespoon of blackstrap molasses
- ½ teaspoon of ginger
- ¼ teaspoon of nutmeg

Directions:

1. Combine the chia seeds with oats and milk in a bowl and mix them well then place them in the fridge for 1 hour.

2. Once the time is up, put all the ingredients in a blender then mix them well until they become smooth.

3. Serve cold and enjoy.

Calories: 478

Peanut Butter and Banana Smoothie

Serves: 3

Ingredients:

- 2 cups of almond milk
- 3 frozen bananas
- 3 tablespoons of natural peanut butter
- 1 tablespoon of chia seeds
- ½ teaspoon of vanilla extract

Directions:

1. Place all the ingredients in a food processor and blend them until they become smooth.

2. Serve it with some ice cubes and enjoy.

Calories: 591

Strawberry and Banana Smoothie

Serves: 1

Ingredients:

- 1 frozen and chopped banana
- 1 cup of frozen strawberries
- 1 cup and half of almond milk
- ¼ cup of frozen blueberries
- 1 table spoon of chia seeds

Directions:

1. In a food processor, blend all the ingredients until they become smooth then serve and enjoy.

Calories: 461

WHY EVERYONE SHOULD CONSIDER GOING PEGAN?

Now that you know all these information about Pegan Diet, you are probably wondering why you should become pegan?

That is so easy, are you on Paleo diet? Are you Vegan? Whether you are Paleo, Vegan or none of them, Pegan Diet is the right diet for you.

Why? That is because Pegan Diet combines 2 of the most efficient and healthier diets in the whole world, which means that you won't have to keep eating plants only and you won't have to consume lots of meat either. Pegan Diet is a perfect balance of the 2 diets as it offers you the best of both of them.

If you want to lose weight in a fast and healthy way, or you simply want to live a healthy life style Pegan Diet fulfils all your desires and exceeds them. Not to mention that it helps you maintain a healthy and perfect body just like you always dreamed of.

SHOPPING LIST

Pegan Diet shopping list is full of ingredients that might seem simple and plain to you, but once you try them in our recipes you will be astonished and bombarded with the explosion of those wonderful flavours.

Here is a list of all the ingredients that you can use for Pegan Diet.

Meat Protein	Plants Protein
Bison	Quinoa
Turkey	Seeds
Venison	Nuts
Eggs	Spirulina
Lamb	Peas
Chicken	Lentils
Grass-fed meat	Beans
Seafood	Nutritional yeast
Fish	
Sweeteners	**Carbohydrates**
Agave nectar	Plantains
Dates	Acorn squash
Dates sugar	Parsnips
Coconut flakes	Wild rice
Coconut nectar	Sweet potatoes
Maple syrup	Winter squash

Fruit juice	Almond flour
Molasses	Quinoa
Cacao powder	Beans
Dry fruits	Brown rice
Dark chocolate	Potatoes
Coconut Sugar	Peas
Honey	Corn
Coconut Syrup	Tapioca
Natural stevia	Black rice
	Noodles shirtaki
	Spaghetti squash
	Lentils
Good Fats	**Beverage**
Sesame oil	Unsweetened almond milk
Avocado oil	Cashew Milk
Avocado	Goat Milk
Macadamia oil	Veggies juice
Coconut oil	Fruits juices
Cashew butter	Coffee
Coconut milk	Wine
Sardines	Coconut water
Goat cheese	
Nuts	

Seeds Almond butter Grass-fed butter Salmon	

Others
Coconut cream , Coconut amino, Vinegar, Veggies broth, Hot chilli sauce, Vanilla extract, Almond flour, Coconut Flour, Goat's milk yogurt, Tapioca flour, Coconut yogurt, Fresh spices, Dry spices, Fish sauce, Mustard, Kelp noodles, Almond meals, Miso.

CONCLUSION

Pegan Diet is a new life style that consists of 2 diets which are Vegan and Paleo diets; which made it more helpful, efficient and better than any other diet.

Pegan Diet might be new, but it is taking its place among the other diets faster each day.

By following Pegan Diet, you get to integrate the best 2 diets in the world in one as well as get only there benefits without any cons.

The best thing about Pegan Diet is that you won't have to spend a lot of money on it; instead it can be accommodated within your finances.

AUTHOR NOTE

Thank you so much for dedicating this time to read my book, it means a lot to me.

After I heard of the Pegan Diet, I could not help myself from thinking that the diet is as efficient as Dr. Mark Hayman said.

But doing so many researches, tried this diet and saw how much efficient it is and really helpful, I decided to write this book to help get more information across in case you want to try it, especially after I noticed that there are not a lot of resources that explain this diet.

Now that you discovered the depths of this miracle diet, you can choose for yourself whether you want to continue as you are, or you want to change your whole life to the best.

Have a Nice Day!

Made in the USA
Middletown, DE
27 July 2015